Reversing Pyoderma Gangrenosum: Kidney Filtration

The Raw Vegan Plant-Based Detoxification & Regeneration Workbook for Healing Patients.

Volume 5

Health Central

Copyright © 2023

Topics Discussed & Journal Structure

Kidney Filtration

Once upon a time, "disease" or dis-ease within the human body did not exist.

Humans lived and passed naturally. It was their ability to live long and healthy lives that allowed for the human race to continue to replicate and evolve. Today we are seeing a different reality unfold.

Our health has become imbalanced because we are no longer consuming the foods intended for us. We are seeing the human body struggle with removing the toxins resulting from this imbalance. This is leading to dysfunction within different locations of the body. Diagnosis of a "disease" follows shortly after.

The location of the dysfunction / dis-ease within your body, whether that is within an organ, gland or nerve, will always stem from the kidneys (and adrenal glands). The key to realise here is that it was a kidney issue before it became a formally labelled "disease".

The kidneys (including the skin) are the main sites where your lymphatic system (the blood washing facility) eliminates its waste and acids. This lymphatic system is your body's sewage system and therefore is responsible for the cleansing of all accumulating waste from tissue and blood.

So when the filtration ability of your kidneys grounds to a halt, your lymphatic system's waste starts to back up and become congested in pockets - this eventually spreads. You now have acids settling into interstitial spaces (in and around the cells) within the tissue.

Any genetic weaknesses that you have inherited will be the first to worsen and develop dis-ease. Extreme environmental factors, such as a mobile phone mast right outside your home – or high levels of hazardous airborne substances, can all play a role in worsening a pre-existing weakness within your body.

In general, we found that the genetically weak tissue that was inherited tends to be the first to be affected before the issue spreads.

Why?

Now that we understand the role of your kidneys and the importance of them filtering well – we move onto the question of why would your kidneys become impaired?

The human body is formed predominantly of liquid. Therefore retaining a healthy level of hydration is an important factor. Based on your consumption, you will alter the chemistry within your body. This will either create a positive environment (hydration) or a negative environment (dehydration).

Your inner chemistry consists of two states – Acidic (pH less than 7) or Basic (Alkaline – pH more than 7). We already acknowledge that acids are damaging and dehydrating - they create a cationic (acidic & congested imbalance) environment within you.

The majority of humans today have strayed away from the raw diet intended for us – with most consuming foods that are resulting in the formation of an acidic chemistry. This applies not only to the food and drink that you consume but also anything that you apply to your skin (creams, lotions, soaps, cosmetics) as this is also ingested.

How?

For your tissue and cells to detoxify, heal and regenerate, you must start to drain your lymphatic system through your kidneys (and skin). This can only be made possible through a change in diet and daily routine.

We must therefore eliminate all low energy, acid and mucus forming foods from our diets (beans, all animal products: meat, dairy, eggs, all processed/frozen foods, wheat/grains: bread, pasta).

Proteins tend to be very straining on the kidneys. Resultantly your body is infiltrated by uric acid and these acids cause the breakdown of your kidneys whilst mucus and stones form.

All of this congestion within the kidneys then causes a significant blockage to the flow of energy through them. Their ability to filter out metabolic waste and toxins is then hindered.

The solution for opening up the kidneys lies with a 100% raw fruit diet, with the occasional vegetables where needed (we found juiced carrots to be extremely healing and regenerative – along with juiced celery – and beetroot).

Herbs

In order to support your kidneys, there are a variety of herbs that can be taken, some of which include: Saw Palmetto, Cleavers, Stinging Nettle, Uva Ursi, Marshmallow Root, Parsley, Dandelion Root, Couch Grass, Corn Silk, Horsetail, Juniper Berries, Goldenrod, Cordyceps.

It should be noted that the adrenal glands and kidneys are very closely related. The adrenal glands sit above the kidneys and produce neurotransmitters that support the activation of kidney filtration. Equally if the kidneys slow down, so do the adrenal glands - they work synergistically (hand-in-hand).

In some cases patients have very weak adrenal glands and this leads to an impaired kidney function. A few factors that can cause weakened adrenal glands include: prolonged stress, toxic environments, and a weak pituitary gland.

Notable herbs that you could use in order to support adrenal gland health include: Sea Kelp, Ashwagandha, Siberian Ginseng, Ho Shou Wu Root, Liquorice Root, Wild Yam Root, Rhodiola.

Fruits offer high astringent (suction on cells/tissue) and hydration value, and they are the most easily digestible foods, with all nutrients being available for fast absorption (providing that the related organs have been cleansed and are functioning as they should be). We have found grapes and all citrus fruits to be highly astringent and cleansing.

Our earliest ancestors lived off the land and as with all other species, ate a predominantly raw diet (mainly fruit with some vegetables). All other species retained their species-specific diet whilst the humans ventured off down the road of excessive cooked and processed foods.

When you return to the diet designed just for you and your species, you will feel your body normalise (hydrate) and balance out (alkalise) as your kidneys re-awaken and rid your body of all the accumulated acids. Your colon will also start to naturally flush itself out.

Real hydration comes through raw living water-dense foods. Cooking out foods destroys this living element and significantly reduces the energy load that the food will provide you – all whilst becoming more energy consuming for your digestive system to process. This is why you feel fatigued after eating a cooked meal – your energy is being used to digest the meal.

Timescales

With your organs (including your adrenal glands and kidneys) having been over-worked and weakened – they will not be functioning as they should be. Your lymphatic system will likely be backed up and in some cases stagnant – and your bowels will also be impeded with mucus, mucoid plaque, biofilms (bacteria, fungi), and parasites plastered on their walls.

Therefore, a key concept to understand is that although you will start to feel a difference relatively quickly – you should be prepared for the longer haul in order to witness the more lasting changes within yourself.

The speed of achieving results can be accelerated with intermittent dry fasting (for 16+ hours) and slow juicing fruit (conserves digestive energy) but equally it should be noted that nothing happens over night – especially when you are healing and reversing years of acidity, dehydration and tissue damage. It is important to manage your own expectations here.

Additionally, the faster the results, the more aggressive the detoxification symptoms will strike, so it is best to find the right balance between fruits and vegetables for more consistent and sustained results. ALWAYS listen to your body at all times and proceed with care.

Everybody reaches their destination in the end after making it into a lifestyle – however long it takes, so do not ever feel pressured to rush at any stage.

The management and conservation of energy within your body is a major contributor of healing. Eating and digesting solid fruit/ vegetable matter uses energy, and this energy could be better used re-directed towards healing and regeneration.

So for extreme cases, we have found intermittent dry fasting for at least 16 hours (always work your way up) – opened with fruit juice (that has been juiced by using a cold press slow juicer) to work well. This is a higher level of detoxification, and with juice, you will experience far more effective nutrient delivery. Note: the "pure" juices sold in supermarkets tend to be pasteurised (pre-heated at high temperatures) and will not have the same benefits as fresh slow-juiced fruit.

Adjust the amount of juice you consume based on how you feel – always listen to your body. It is easy for practitioners to recommend drinking 3 to 5 litres of juice to all patients but in reality, everybody is different and there are too many factors involved to make such a generalised recommendation. Factors such as: age, height, weight, body fat percentage, body type, current organ weaknesses.

With patients that were not in a critical state, we recommended a slower transition into a fruit diet – with some vegetables/salads where necessary. Once fully raw vegan, our goal was to maintain their routine for a month or two before introducing intermittent dry fasting. The fasting supported an improvement in kidney filtration – and this allowed for an increase in acidic waste to be drained out from the body. Remember to always keep up water intake after any type of fasting.

The skin (known as the 3rd kidney) can also drain your lymphatic system's waste through deep sweat (sauna or even better; a hot climate) – contributing to the fight against systemic acidosis.

Open up all of your kidneys and filtration channels - and you will soon witness the positive changes that you desire.

Your Notes & Thoughts

Main takeaways from this section. Any realisations?
Actions to take. *Why is healing important to you?* What
are you looking forward to?

Our Story

It was a Sunday night, over 7 years ago – I was in bed – tossing and turning – unable to sleep. I watched the time pass, from 11pm, to 12am… to 1:30am. I just couldn't sleep. I could feel an immense pressure in my chest cavity and all across my diaphragm area. I couldn't understand where this was coming from. I got up and had some water, I then tried to use the bathroom – the discomfort was still there. Nothing seemed to work – I felt like I was being suffocated each time I would lie down. In the end, I fell asleep out of sheer fatigue.

At the time, I was a sufferer of asthma, eczema, anxiety attacks, and a damaged/leaky gut. These conditions had lead to many symptoms that doctors could not offer me any answers for. I had many tests done but nothing could tell me what the root causes of my problems were.

I started researching about my symptoms, and as I did this, I found myself expanding into the area of medical history. As my research continued, I came to understand that our ancestors lived healthy and long lives, without the health challenges of today.

Eventually, I stumbled upon a few health forums which I joined. Through these, I met a series of individuals that were battling a variety of conditions themselves (a rare genetic disorder, Crohn's disease, multiple sclerosis, muscular dystrophy (MD), diabetes, cushing's disease, a series of 'incurable' autoimmune diseases, and cancer).

We all came together and as we started to grow as a group, we made a significant discovery - that actually the cure to all diseases was discovered back in the 1920s by a Dr Arnold Ehret.

As we studied his material, we started applying his information and protocols on ourselves. This seemed like one experiment worth trying, and within 2 weeks, regardless of our individual conditions, we all started to notice a difference in our improved digestion, higher energy levels, increased mental clarity and improved physical ability. A major change was taking place – our health was improving, as our conditions were decreasing.

We continued to expand our knowledge and we started to encounter even more communities and learnt that there were more magnificent and very gifted healers out there. We came across the works and achievements of Dr Sebi, and completed an insightful and very informative course by Dr Robert Morse.

The essential message of these great healers was very similar to that of Dr Arnold Ehret. Now we had even further confirmation that the information we had been following thus far was in fact THE path to health success. With our progress so far, we could sense victory.

Within 3 months, 30 to 40 percent of our symptoms had disappeared and our health was becoming stronger. Some of us started to take specific herbs in order to enhance the detoxification.

Another 3 months on and the majority of us no longer experienced any more symptoms. Our blood work had also improved significantly, but we still had work to do in order to completely heal.

Now that we had made significant progress in reversing our conditions through self-experimentation, we started to offer basic healthy eating advice to the sick within our local communities.

Eventually, we started working with local patients on a voluntary basis. It was heartbreaking to witness lives being cut short or chronic sickness being accepted as a way of life – all whilst the lifelong eating habits of these individuals remained. The most common diseases that we were coming across included: cancers, heart disease, chronic kidney disease, high blood pressure, varying infections, and diabetes.

By helping our communities with changing their daily eating habits, we started seeing results, and although the transitional phase of moving from the foods that they were so used to eating, to moving over to a raw plant-based routine was a challenge, in the end, it was worth the shift. Note: there were many that ignored our advice and sadly they continued to remain in their state.

We did have resistance initially from family members and friends of the sick but after some time as they started seeing health improvements, more started joining us, and they also started experiencing what we had when we first set out on our journey of natural self-healing.

Nevertheless, challenges still remained – the main ones being the undoing of society's programming that cooked food is an essential part of life (including animal and wheat based products) and raw food alone surely cannot be good for you. It doesn't take long to explain how to remove imbalances and dis-ease from within the human body but the more extensive task is to actually have the protocol information applied and adhered to completely.

This is where the idea for this series of journal & progress tracker stemmed from. We felt compelled to spread this information in a more digestible and applicable form, over a series of volumes, in which we would start by offering some key informative points, followed by a journal which would allow for you to actually apply the information, record your progress, daily feelings and stay accountable to yourself. We also found that journaling and writing to oneself really helps to self-motivate and enhances a self consciousness that is needed when following a protocol like this.

Each journal volume within this series will be designed to help you record your journey for a 30 day period. At the start of each journal we will continue to offer insightful information about our experiences, whilst expanding on and re-iterating specific parts of this protocol.

The fact that you are reading this foreword is an indication that you are already on your way to self-healing. Regardless of your condition, we invite you to seek more knowledge and set your health free.

May you always remain blessed and guided.

Much Love From The Health Central Team

Important Notes for Overcoming Your Pyoderma Gangrenosum

1. It should be noted that based on our experiences and understanding, whether your condition is Pyoderma Gangrenosum, or any other, we recommend the same raw vegan healing protocol across all spectrums. With some conditions, you may need to perform a deeper detoxification (using herbs - or organ/glandular meat/capsules for more chronic situations) before achieving significant results, but in general, we have found this protocol to work in most cases. In our experience, the goal is not to cure, but instead to raise health levels first, through healthy food choices, as intended for our species – before the eradication and prevention of these modern-day "disease" conditions can take place.

2. With all conditions, we have found that the lymphatic system has become congested and overwhelmed due to the kidneys not efficiently filtering out the accumulated cell waste – as a result of years of dehydrating cooked/wheat/dairy foods. The adrenal glands work closely with the kidneys, and so adrenal/kidney herbs and glandular formulas played a major role in opening up these channels. We also found that opening up the bowels and loosening the gut was hugely important too.

3. The healing protocol that we used on ourselves is discussed and expanded upon throughout the various volumes in this series. Our goal is to share information that we have gathered from our journeys, and let you decide if it is something that you feel could also work for you in your

journey for health and vitality. You are not obliged to use this information, and you may proceed as you see fit.

Through our study, research and application, we have found this system to correct any internal imbalances and remove dis-ease that has occurred within the human body, due to the continued consumption of acid-forming foods.

4. Always take progression ultra slow and go at your own pace. Listen to your body at every stage. We cannot re-iterate this point enough. Pay attention to how you feel and continue to consult your doctor and monitor your blood work.

5. A special emphasis needs to be given to the transition phase when moving from your regular, standard diet, to a raw vegan diet that is high in fruit. You must take your time and slowly remove foods from your current routine, and replace them with either fasting or a small amount of fruit in the initial stages. Work with small amounts – please do not make any drastic changes. If you do not feel comfortable or have any concerns at any stage, please immediately stop.

Note: with any dietary change, this can be a stressful event for the body and so it is important that you support your kidneys and adrenal glands using the appropriate herbs and glandular formulas previously mentioned.

6. Before partaking in any new dietary routine, please always consult your Doctor first and ensure that they are aware of your health related goals. This approach is beneficial because (a) you can monitor your blood work with your doctor as you progress with this new protocol, and (b) if you are on any medication, as your health improves, you

can review its need and/or discuss having dosage amounts reduced (if necessary).

7. Please note that we are sharing information from our collective experiences of how we healed ourselves from a variety of diseases and conditions. These are solely our own opinions. Having reversed a range of conditions using essentially the same protocol, our understanding and conclusion, based on our experience alone, is that regardless of the disease, illness or condition name – removing it from the human body stems from correcting your diet and transitioning over to a more raw vegan lifestyle.

8. Proceed with care, and again, do not make any sudden changes – always take your time in slowly removing foods that are not serving you, and replacing them with high energy sweet tree-ripened juicy fruit. If at any point you feel that you are moving too quickly, please adjust your transition accordingly. Results may vary between individuals.

9. We recommended that you constantly expand your knowledge and familiarise yourself with the works of Dr Arnold Ehret, Dr Robert Morse and John Rose. When you feel confident with your understanding, start taking gradual steps towards reaching your goals. Make the most of this journal and use it to serve you as a companion on your journey.

The Power of Journaling

a) Journaling your inner self talk is a truly effective way of increasing self awareness and consciousness. To be able to transfer your thoughts and feelings onto a piece of paper is a truly effective method of self reflection and improvement. This is much needed when you are switching to a high fruit dietary routine.

b) Be sure to always add the date of journaling at the top of each page used. This is invaluable for when you wish to go back and review/track progress and your feelings/thoughts on previous dates.

c) Keep a comprehensive record of activities, thoughts, and really log everything you ate/are eating. You can even make miscellaneous notes if you feel that they will help you.

d) We have added tips and questions to offer you guidance, reminders, inspiration and areas to journal about.

e) We like to use journals to have a conversation with ourselves. Inner talk can really help you overcome any challenges that you are experiencing. Express yourself and any concerns that you may have.

f) Try to advise yourself as though you are your best friend – similarly to how you would advise a close friend or family member. You will be surprised at the results that you will achieve from using this technique.

g) Add notes to this journal and work your way through the 30 days. Once completed, move onto the next journal volume in this series, which will also be structured in a similar, supportive and educational fashion. We have produced a series of these journals in order to cater for your ongoing journey and goals.

h) For those of you who would like to track your progress with a more basic notebook-style journal, we have produced a separate series in which each notebook interior differs. This is to cater for your complete health journaling needs.

We have laid out the following examples to serve as potential frameworks for one way of how a journal could be filled in on a daily basis. These are just basic examples, but you can complete your daily journals in any other way that you feel is most comfortable and effective for you.

[EXAMPLE 1]
Today's Date: 2nd Jan 2020

Morning

I just ate 3 mangoes - very sweet and tasty. I felt a heavy feeling under my chest area so I stopped eating. Unsure what that was - maybe digestive or the transverse colon?

Afternoon

I was feeling hungry so I am eating some dried figs, pineapple and apricots with around 750ml of spring water.

Evening

Sipping on a green tea (herbal). Feeling pretty strong and alert at the moment.

Night

Enjoying a bowl of red seeded grapes. Currently I feel satisfied.

Today's Notes (Highlights, Thoughts, Feelings):

Unlike yesterday, today was a good day. I am noticing an increase in regular bowel movements which makes me feel cleansed and light afterwards. I feel as though my kidneys are also starting to filter better (white sediment visible in morning wee).

It definitely helps to document my thoughts in this workbook. A great way to reflect, improve and stay on track.

Feeling very good - vibrant and strong - I have noticed a major improvement in my physical fitness and performance. Mentally I feel healthier and happier.

Today's Date: 3rd Jan 2020

Morning

Dry fasting (water and food free since 8pm last night) - will go up until 12:30pm today, and start with 500ml of spring water before eating half a watermelon.

Afternoon

Kept busy and was in and out quite a bit – so nothing consumed.

Evening

At around 5pm, I had a peppermint tea with a selection of mixed dried fruit (small bowl of apricot, dates, mango, pineapple, and prunes).

Night

Sipped on spring water through the evening as required.
Finished off the other half of the watermelon from the morning.

Today's Notes (Highlights, Thoughts, Feelings):

As with most days, today started well with me dry fasting (continuing my fast from my sleep/skipping breakfast) up until around 12:30pm and then eating half a watermelon. The laxative effect of the watermelon helped me poop and release any loosened toxins from the fasting period.
I tend to struggle on some days from 3pm onwards. Up until that point I am okay but if the cravings strike then it can be challenging. I remind myself that those burgers and chips do not have any live healing energy.
I feel good in general. I feel fantastic doing a fruit/juice fast but slightly empty by the end of the day.
Cooked food makes me feel severe fatigue and mental fog.
Will continue with my fruit fasting and start to introduce fruit juices due to their deeper detox benefits. I would love to be on juices only as I have seen others within the community achieve amazing results.

[EXAMPLE 3]

Today's Date: 4th Jan 2020

Morning

Today I woke and my children were enjoying some watermelon for breakfast – and the smell was luring so I joined them. Large bowl of watermelon eaten at around 8am. Started with a glass of water.

Afternoon

Snacked on left over watermelon throughout the morning and afternoon. Had 5 dates an hour or so after.

Evening

Had around 3 mangoes at around 6pm. Felt content – but then I was invited round to a family gathering where a selection of pizzas, burgers and chips were being served. I gave into the peer pressure and felt like I let myself down!

Night

Having over-eaten earlier on in the evening, I was still feeling bloated with a headache (possibly digestion related) and I also felt quite mucus filled (wheez in chest and coughing up phlegm). Very sleepy and low energy. The perils of cooked foods!!

Today's Notes (Highlights, Thoughts, Feelings):

I let myself down today. It all started well until I ate a fully blown meal (and over-ate). I didn't remain focussed and I spun off track. As a result my energy levels were much lower and I felt a bout of extreme fatigue 30 minutes after the meal (most likely the body struggling to with digesting all that cooked food).

I need to stick to the plan because the difference between fruit fasting, and eating cooked foods is huge – 1 makes you feel empowered whilst the other makes you feel drained. I also felt the mucus overload after the meal – it kicked in pretty quickly.

Today I felt disappointed after giving in to the meal but tomorrow is a new day and I will keep on going! It is important to remind myself that I won't get better if I cannot stick to the routine.

Frequently Asked Questions (Vol. 5)

1. Will this really work for me?

Yes. We are sent this question quite often. The reason why the prospect of eating a high fruit raw diet is so daunting and strange to us is because we have been so heavily brainwashed by the norms of society. Advertising of the latest food trends has hypnotised us and so we are no longer able to see through our self-formed reality. Our family's eating trends also play a role in our belief that we must eat in a certain way. Social eating is another major contributor to this. Eating from the land is the diet intended for our species. As children, we were naturally attracted towards fruit over cooked foods. However, the only way to develop belief in this way of eating is to experience its benefits first-hand – try eating a fruit-only diet of your favourite fruit for 5 days, and take a note of; how you feel, your sleep quality, your energy levels, mental clarity, digestion and elimination – you're welcome to give it a go. You will come to your own conclusions at this point.

2. Will your other book volumes help me?

Yes. We have covered a variety of unique topics in the different book volumes found in this series. Each is geared around educating and supporting you in reaching your goals of good health and being "disease" free. When you are moving from years of eating a mucus-forming diet - to eating fully raw - you should be informed about the different aspects of the new protocol. There are many areas and angles within the scope of healing and normalising your body's state and ridding it of "disease".

Not everything can be covered in one volume. You will also find different Frequently Asked Questions (sent in to us by our readers) in each book and these question-and-answer sections are also very insightful and helpful. In summary, the different book volumes will guide and support you through your healing journey whilst offering you encouragement.

3. My MD (Medical Doctor) is encouraging me to stick to my current diet and medication schedule. What should I do?

This is a very good question as it is a common topic that we face on a regular basis. We do not advise you to stop taking your medicines. We are offering our insights and experience into the healing benefits that we have witnessed firsthand as a result of applying this protocol to ourselves and our patients. This raw vegan protocol is geared around slowly transitioning to a predominantly fruit diet with some vegetables and salads to accompany. It is important to assure your MD that you will continue to take the prescribed medicines as part of your new dietary routine. We do advise working closely with your MD. Ask to have a review of your medicines each time you feel differently within, because as your health improves and you strengthen, you will inevitably require less medication. Keep in mind that MDs may not be trained in nutrition and healing – but more so on medicines and symptom management. Cure yourself and become the example for others to learn from.

1. Today's Date:

Morning
(work towards continuing your night time dry fast up until at least 12pm)

Afternoon
(get hydrating with fresh fruit or even better slow juiced fruits/berries/melons)

Evening
(aim to wind down to a dry fast by around 6pm to 7pm)

Night
(work your way up to dry fasting from the evening until 12pm the following day)

Today's Notes (Highlights, Thoughts, Feelings, What Could You Improve On?)

"Get yourself an accountability partner to complete a 30 day detox with. Start with 7 days and work your way up. It will be fun and motivating completing it with somebody (or a group) ...or of course you can go it alone."

---

2. Today's Date:

Morning
(work towards continuing your night time dry fast up until at least 12pm)

Afternoon
(get hydrating with fresh fruit or even better slow juiced fruits/berries/melons)

Evening
(aim to wind down to a dry fast by around 6pm to 7pm)

Night
(work your way up to dry fasting from the evening until 12pm the following day)

Today's Notes (Highlights, Thoughts, Feelings, What Could You Improve On?)

"Remember when starting out, it is important to keep yourself hydrated throughout the day. Spring Water is a good start - and slow/cold pressed juice is also very powerful."

3. Today's Date:

————————————— Morning —————————————
(work towards continuing your night time dry fast up until at least 12pm)

————————————— Afternoon —————————————
(get hydrating with fresh fruit or even better slow juiced fruits/berries/melons)

————————————— Evening —————————————
(aim to wind down to a dry fast by around 6pm to 7pm)

————————————— Night —————————————
(work your way up to dry fasting from the evening until 12pm the following day)

Today's Notes (Highlights, Thoughts, Feelings, What Could You Improve On?)

"Eat melons/watermelons separately, and before any other fruit as it digests faster and we want to limit fermentation (acidity) which can occur if other fruits are mixed in."

4. Today's Date:

Morning
(work towards continuing your night time dry fast up until at least 12pm)

Afternoon
(get hydrating with fresh fruit or even better slow juiced fruits/berries/melons)

Evening
(aim to wind down to a dry fast by around 6pm to 7pm)

Night
(work your way up to dry fasting from the evening until 12pm the following day)

Today's Notes (Highlights, Thoughts, Feelings, What Could You Improve On?)

"Stay focussed on the end goal of removing mucus & toxins from your body and feeling wonderful! Look forward to being full of vitality and disease free once again"

5. Today's Date:

———————— Morning ————————
(work towards continuing your night time dry fast up until at least 12pm)

———————— Afternoon ————————
(get hydrating with fresh fruit or even better slow juiced fruits/berries/melons)

———————— Evening ————————
(aim to wind down to a dry fast by around 6pm to 7pm)

———————— Night ————————
(work your way up to dry fasting from the evening until 12pm the following day)

Today's Notes (Highlights, Thoughts, Feelings, What Could You Improve On?)

"Meditate and perform deep breathing exercises in order to help yourself remain present minded and on track. Perform these techniques throughout the day but also during any challenging times that you may come to face."

6. Today's Date:

Morning
(work towards continuing your night time dry fast up until at least 12pm)

Afternoon
(get hydrating with fresh fruit or even better slow juiced fruits/berries/melons)

Evening
(aim to wind down to a dry fast by around 6pm to 7pm)

Night
(work your way up to dry fasting from the evening until 12pm the following day)

Today's Notes (Highlights, Thoughts, Feelings, What Could You Improve On?)

"Join a few like-minded communities – there are many juicing and raw vegan based groups, both online and offline. Being part of a community can help motivate you to reach your goals. You will also learn a great amount from others. Seeing others succeed is empowering."

---

7. Today's Date:

Morning
(work towards continuing your night time dry fast up until at least 12pm)

Afternoon
(get hydrating with fresh fruit or even better slow juiced fruits/berries/melons)

Evening
(aim to wind down to a dry fast by around 6pm to 7pm)

Night
(work your way up to dry fasting from the evening until 12pm the following day)

Today's Notes (Highlights, Thoughts, Feelings, What Could You Improve On?)

"If you are struggling to cope with hunger pangs in the early stages, try some dates or dried apricots, prunes, or raisins, with a cup of herbal tea. However, these pangs will disappear once your body adjusts to your new routine."

8. Today's Date:

—————————— Morning ——————————
(work towards continuing your night time dry fast up until at least 12pm)

—————————— Afternoon ——————————
(get hydrating with fresh fruit or even better slow juiced fruits/berries/melons)

—————————— Evening ——————————
(aim to wind down to a dry fast by around 6pm to 7pm)

—————————— Night ——————————
(work your way up to dry fasting from the evening until 12pm the following day)

Today's Notes (Highlights, Thoughts, Feelings, What Could You Improve On?)

"Get into a routine of regularly buying fresh fruit (or grow your own if weather permits) to keep your supplies up. Local wholesale markets do also clear fruits/veg on Fridays (if they are closed for the weekend) at a lower price, so they are worth a visit."

9. Today's Date:

Morning
(work towards continuing your night time dry fast up until at least 12pm)

Afternoon
(get hydrating with fresh fruit or even better slow juiced fruits/berries/melons)

Evening
(aim to wind down to a dry fast by around 6pm to 7pm)

Night
(work your way up to dry fasting from the evening until 12pm the following day)

Today's Notes (Highlights, Thoughts, Feelings, What Could You Improve On?)

"Regularly remind yourself about the great rewards and benefits that you will experience by keeping up this detoxification process. Imagine the lives you could save as a result of healing yourself."

10. Today's Date:

—————————— Morning ——————————
(work towards continuing your night time dry fast up until at least 12pm)

—————————— Afternoon ——————————
(get hydrating with fresh fruit or even better slow juiced fruits/berries/melons)

—————————— Evening ——————————
(aim to wind down to a dry fast by around 6pm to 7pm)

—————————— Night ——————————
(work your way up to dry fasting from the evening until 12pm the following day)

Today's Notes (Highlights, Thoughts, Feelings, What Could You Improve On?)

"Keep your teeth brushed (using miswak; a natural brush). Use coconut oil to oil pull before bedtime. Done correctly, you will notice an improvement in your dental health with these practices."

11. Today's Date:

Morning

(work towards continuing your night time dry fast up until at least 12pm)

Afternoon

(get hydrating with fresh fruit or even better slow juiced fruits/berries/melons)

Evening

(aim to wind down to a dry fast by around 6pm to 7pm)

Night

(work your way up to dry fasting from the evening until 12pm the following day)

Today's Notes (Highlights, Thoughts, Feelings, What Could You Improve On?)

"Be motivated by the vision of becoming an example for others to learn from and follow. You could change the lives of family and friends by showing them your own improvements."

12. Today's Date:

Morning
(work towards continuing your night time dry fast up until at least 12pm)

Afternoon
(get hydrating with fresh fruit or even better slow juiced fruits/berries/melons)

Evening
(aim to wind down to a dry fast by around 6pm to 7pm)

Night
(work your way up to dry fasting from the evening until 12pm the following day)

Today's Notes (Highlights, Thoughts, Feelings, What Could You Improve On?)

"Embrace your achievements and wonderful results – feel and appreciate the difference within you as a result of this new routine. Notice how your personal agility and fitness has improved. Feel the improved energy levels."

13. Today's Date:

Morning
(work towards continuing your night time dry fast up until at least 12pm)

Afternoon
(get hydrating with fresh fruit or even better slow juiced fruits/berries/melons)

Evening
(aim to wind down to a dry fast by around 6pm to 7pm)

Night
(work your way up to dry fasting from the evening until 12pm the following day)

Today's Notes (Highlights, Thoughts, Feelings, What Could You Improve On?)

*"Buy fruit in bulk where possible so you have
ample supplies for a week or two in advance.
If in a hot climate, you could even freeze your
fruit or make ice lollies out of it (crush & freeze).
Immerse yourself in fruit so it becomes your only option."*

14. Today's Date:

Morning
(work towards continuing your night time dry fast up until at least 12pm)

Afternoon
(get hydrating with fresh fruit or even better slow juiced fruits/berries/melons)

Evening
(aim to wind down to a dry fast by around 6pm to 7pm)

Night
(work your way up to dry fasting from the evening until 12pm the following day)

Today's Notes (Highlights, Thoughts, Feelings, What Could You Improve On?)

"Stay as busy as you can during the daytime. Creating a busy routine makes it easier to manage your diet. Have a purpose, and keep setting yourself new tasks/actions in order to keep yourself occupied."

15. Today's Date:

Morning
(work towards continuing your night time dry fast up until at least 12pm)

Afternoon
(get hydrating with fresh fruit or even better slow juiced fruits/berries/melons)

Evening
(aim to wind down to a dry fast by around 6pm to 7pm)

Night
(work your way up to dry fasting from the evening until 12pm the following day)

Today's Notes (Highlights, Thoughts, Feelings, What Could You Improve On?)

"Complete your fruit and fasting routine with a group of friends/family/colleagues so you can all support one another. Make it fun - set challenges - dry fast together and break your fasts together - have weekly catch up sessions."

16. Today's Date:

Morning
(work towards continuing your night time dry fast up until at least 12pm)

Afternoon
(get hydrating with fresh fruit or even better slow juiced fruits/berries/melons)

Evening
(aim to wind down to a dry fast by around 6pm to 7pm)

Night
(work your way up to dry fasting from the evening until 12pm the following day)

Today's Notes (Highlights, Thoughts, Feelings, What Could You Improve On?)

"Look out for white cloud/sediment (acids) in your urine to confirm that your kidneys are filtering out waste. Urinate in a glass jar - leave for 2 hours to settle before observing."

17. Today's Date:

Morning
(work towards continuing your night time dry fast up until at least 12pm)

Afternoon
(get hydrating with fresh fruit or even better slow juiced fruits/berries/melons)

Evening
(aim to wind down to a dry fast by around 6pm to 7pm)

Night
(work your way up to dry fasting from the evening until 12pm the following day)

Today's Notes (Highlights, Thoughts, Feelings, What Could You Improve On?)

"Have genuine love and care for yourself. If you are craving junk food, affirm positive inner talk ("I won't feel good after eating junk. I love myself too much to put my body through that - so leave it out!"). You can also take Sea Kelp, Coconut Water, or Celery to reduce any salt cravings."

18. Today's Date:

——————————— Morning ———————————
(work towards continuing your night time dry fast up until at least 12pm)

——————————— Afternoon ———————————
(get hydrating with fresh fruit or even better slow juiced fruits/berries/melons)

——————————— Evening ———————————
(aim to wind down to a dry fast by around 6pm to 7pm)

——————————— Night ———————————
(work your way up to dry fasting from the evening until 12pm the following day)

Today's Notes (Highlights, Thoughts, Feelings, What Could You Improve On?)

"Feel and note down the difference within yourself as you filter out unwanted acids with this alkaline, water-dense high fruit protocol."

19. Today's Date:

Morning
(work towards continuing your night time dry fast up until at least 12pm)

Afternoon
(get hydrating with fresh fruit or even better slow juiced fruits/berries/melons)

Evening
(aim to wind down to a dry fast by around 6pm to 7pm)

Night
(work your way up to dry fasting from the evening until 12pm the following day)

Today's Notes (Highlights, Thoughts, Feelings, What Could You Improve On?)

"Look for acidic waste/sediments in your urine regularly in order to ensure your kidneys are filtering. Dry fasting for over 18 hours will increase kidney filtration. You can also drink the juice of slow-juiced citrus fruits (lemons, oranges). Sweating helps too."

20. Today's Date:

Morning

(work towards continuing your night time dry fast up until at least 12pm)

Afternoon

(get hydrating with fresh fruit or even better slow juiced fruits/berries/melons)

Evening

(aim to wind down to a dry fast by around 6pm to 7pm)

Night

(work your way up to dry fasting from the evening until 12pm the following day)

Today's Notes (Highlights, Thoughts, Feelings, What Could You Improve On?)

"Infections emerge in an acidic environment. In order to remove infections, you must concentrate on kidney filtration. Use herbs for kidneys and adrenal glands - using dry fasting to assist."

21. Today's Date:

Morning

(work towards continuing your night time dry fast up until at least 12pm)

Afternoon

(get hydrating with fresh fruit or even better slow juiced fruits/berries/melons)

Evening

(aim to wind down to a dry fast by around 6pm to 7pm)

Night

(work your way up to dry fasting from the evening until 12pm the following day)

Today's Notes (Highlights, Thoughts, Feelings, What Could You Improve On?)

"Any deficiencies that you may have will start to disappear once you have cleansed your congested gut/colon, kidneys and various other eliminative organs."

22. Today's Date:

Morning

(work towards continuing your night time dry fast up until at least 12pm)

Afternoon

(get hydrating with fresh fruit or even better slow juiced fruits/berries/melons)

Evening

(aim to wind down to a dry fast by around 6pm to 7pm)

Night

(work your way up to dry fasting from the evening until 12pm the following day)

Today's Notes (Highlights, Thoughts, Feelings, What Could You Improve On?)

"Dependant on how deeply you detoxify yourself, it is possible to eliminate any genetic weaknesses that you may have inherited. This will require a deep detoxification process which involves juicing your fruits with prolonged periods of dry fasting"

---

23. Today's Date:

Morning
(work towards continuing your night time dry fast up until at least 12pm)

Afternoon
(get hydrating with fresh fruit or even better slow juiced fruits/berries/melons)

Evening
(aim to wind down to a dry fast by around 6pm to 7pm)

Night
(work your way up to dry fasting from the evening until 12pm the following day)

Today's Notes (Highlights, Thoughts, Feelings, What Could You Improve On?)

"Stay focused on your detoxification for deeper, lasting results. All past injuries / trauma are also repairable for good. Get those old acids out and replace them with a pain-free alkaline environment"

24. Today's Date:

Morning

(work towards continuing your night time dry fast up until at least 12pm)

Afternoon

(get hydrating with fresh fruit or even better slow juiced fruits/berries/melons)

Evening

(aim to wind down to a dry fast by around 6pm to 7pm)

Night

(work your way up to dry fasting from the evening until 12pm the following day)

Today's Notes (Highlights, Thoughts, Feelings, What Could You Improve On?)

*"If you suffer from ongoing sadness / depression, a deep detox will support your mental health. You will soon notice a positive change in your mood. **Note:** you will need to support your adrenal glands and kidneys with glandulars and/or herbs (liqorice root, sea kelp, uva ursi, nettle)"*

25. Today's Date:

Morning
(work towards continuing your night time dry fast up until at least 12pm)

Afternoon
(get hydrating with fresh fruit or even better slow juiced fruits/berries/melons)

Evening
(aim to wind down to a dry fast by around 6pm to 7pm)

Night
(work your way up to dry fasting from the evening until 12pm the following day)

Today's Notes (Highlights, Thoughts, Feelings, What Could You Improve On?)

"Have your fruits/ juices throughout the day - with dry fasting gaps of at least 3 hours in-between each feed. As the evening approaches, start to dry fast fully – from this point on, your body wants to rest and heal."

26. Today's Date:

Morning
(work towards continuing your night time dry fast up until at least 12pm)

Afternoon
(get hydrating with fresh fruit or even better slow juiced fruits/berries/melons)

Evening
(aim to wind down to a dry fast by around 6pm to 7pm)

Night
(work your way up to dry fasting from the evening until 12pm the following day)

Today's Notes (Highlights, Thoughts, Feelings, What Could You Improve On?)

"The kidneys dislike proteins but really appreciate juicy fruits like melons, berries, citrus fruits, pineapples, mangoes, apples, grapes. Witness the difference by replacing cooked foods and protein with fruits. Become the change."

27. Today's Date:

Morning
(work towards continuing your night time dry fast up until at least 12pm)

Afternoon
(get hydrating with fresh fruit or even better slow juiced fruits/berries/melons)

Evening
(aim to wind down to a dry fast by around 6pm to 7pm)

Night
(work your way up to dry fasting from the evening until 12pm the following day)

Today's Notes (Highlights, Thoughts, Feelings, What Could You Improve On?)

"Healing is very easy. There's no need to complicate it. Keep everything simple and you will see results. Concentrate on improving your level of health to a point where dis-ease is dissolved"

28. Today's Date:

Morning
(work towards continuing your night time dry fast up until at least 12pm)

Afternoon
(get hydrating with fresh fruit or even better slow juiced fruits/berries/melons)

Evening
(aim to wind down to a dry fast by around 6pm to 7pm)

Night
(work your way up to dry fasting from the evening until 12pm the following day)

Today's Notes (Highlights, Thoughts, Feelings, What Could You Improve On?)

"Keep your body in an alkaline and hydrated state as this is where regeneration takes place - and disease cannot continue to exist. You can achieve this through a raw fruits and vegetables diet (find your balance between the two)"

29. Today's Date:

———————— Morning ————————
(work towards continuing your night time dry fast up until at least 12pm)

———————— Afternoon ————————
(get hydrating with fresh fruit or even better slow juiced fruits/berries/melons)

———————— Evening ————————
(aim to wind down to a dry fast by around 6pm to 7pm)

———————— Night ————————
(work your way up to dry fasting from the evening until 12pm the following day)

Today's Notes (Highlights, Thoughts, Feelings, What Could You Improve On?)

"An enema with boiled water (cooled down) can support your detox. However this high fruit dietary protocol will encourage healthy bowel movement and this should be sufficient, unless if you are at a chronic stage."

30. Today's Date:

Morning
(work towards continuing your night time dry fast up until at least 12pm)

Afternoon
(get hydrating with fresh fruit or even better slow juiced fruits/berries/melons)

Evening
(aim to wind down to a dry fast by around 6pm to 7pm)

Night
(work your way up to dry fasting from the evening until 12pm the following day)

Today's Notes (Highlights, Thoughts, Feelings, What Could You Improve On?)

"You can have your iris' read by an iridologist that works with Dr Bernard Jensen's system. An Iris Diagnosis will offer you information on specific areas of weakness that pre-exist for you to focus on."

.

www.ingramcontent.com/pod-product-compliance
Lightning Source LLC
Chambersburg PA
CBHW031204020426
42333CB00013B/792